5 STEPS to a PAIN-FREE BACK & NECK

How to Get Instant, Lasting Relief Without Drugs or Surgery...So You Enjoy a Pain-Free Life!

Michael Greenspan

Testimonials

"I have been coming to The Back and Neck Relief Center for several years (2007) and I love it! Every therapist is professional, knowledgeable, and skilled. These are the best treatments I have ever gotten and help relieve pain from everyday stress and workouts. I get a treatment every weekend, and the prices are great too!" - Marilyn Mobey, Manhattan Beach

"The treatments at The Back and Neck Relief Center are the only thing that has helped with my neck and shoulder pain. I have severe muscle spasms and when I leave here, I feel relaxed and pain-free." - Tina, Long Beach

"The Back and Neck Relief Center rocks! The quality of the therapists is fantastic- always feel amazing afterwards!! The scheduling is always so easy and friendly. Love the reminder calls! Thank you for everything- love you guys!!" - Lori DeFelice, Los Angeles

"I was suffering from pain in ligaments around the tailbone and lower back area. The Back and Neck Relief Center's therapists worked hard to relieve the tension carried in my shoulders and neck because of this condition. I'm feeling so much better!" - Dawn Robinson, Manhattan Beach

"I started treatment care at The Back and Neck Relief Center in May 2015 with low back, neck pain, headaches, Achilles tendonitis, and sciatica for the past three years. I saw two doctors, three other massage therapists, and 1 physical therapist. My life was interrupted competing as an athlete… my ability to compete at a high level was non-existent until beginning my therapy at The Back and Neck Relief Center. The balance of consistent therapy allowed me to return to the track to compete at the Military World Championship and a number of other international competitions. The neuromuscular treatments provided at The Back and Neck Relief Center are second to none." - Manny Smith, Hermosa Beach

"I started at The Back and Neck Relief Center in April 2014. I do therapy not because of ailments but as general maintenance. I am a very active senior citizen so I use this therapy to get the knots out, the muscles smooth and the joints loose. I do a 1 ½ hour deep tissue treatment every week… When I skip a visit, I can feel the difference. I have been doing weekly treatments for 15 years, and I am convinced that it allows me to regularly play tennis, power walk for a distance and workout at the gym, without joint pain or muscle soreness not related to overuse. I generally sleep well and move around on the court way better than my peers.
I find The Back and Neck Relief Center therapists to be very competent, knowledgeable, friendly, and responsive to my needs. I regularly use three therapists in a weekly rotation. As each has

different strengths, i.e.; back, legs, etc., I get all of the parts fully attended to and I feel great. P.S: I am 81 years old." - PE Dorr

"I started coming to The Back and Neck Relief Center 1/13/19 for knee pain and Achilles pain, that I had for 3 years. I saw 6 other practitioners for help, 1 M.D., 3 PT's, UCLA surgery dept. (I didn't have surgery) and a chiropractor. My normal life was interrupted due to chronic pain, limiting physical activities but avoiding those activities led to weakness and tightness. In 5 treatments or so, results became apparent. Treatments from The Back and Neck Relief Center have helped me begin to overcome tightness that has contributed to my knee and achilles pain. Two therapists in particular made an immediate impact. They are very skilled and my pain has been significantly reduced. They were also great at communicating with me about how my muscles felt so that I could focus on things like foam rolling between treatments." - Jane Evans, Culver City

"The most amazing therapist helped me feel better than I have in a long time! The tension is gone and I feel lighter and healthier in my body!!! Fantastic- can't wait to get back!" - Caryn Richman, Manhattan Beach

"My shoulders and calves were tense and stiff prior to my visit. My therapist had some great pointers for improving my posture and she worked magic..." - Yukari Tanimoto, Palos Verdes Peninsula

"My neck and shoulders were getting so stiff that I was having trouble turning my head from side to side. My shoulders were always slumped and sore. With the weekly treatments here at The Back and Neck Relief Center, I feel more limber and the muscles are supple." - Karen Sugita, Manhattan Beach

"The Back and Neck Relief Center has been a great find. Their team of experienced therapists have been so great from the beginning and continue to provide very great service. I recommend them to anyone who is looking to alleviate stress, pain, or who just wants to relax." - Ruth Gallo, Manhattan Beach

"I've been coming to The Back and Neck Relief Center for the past 6 months with degenerative disk disease, neck and back pain, and muscle spasms, that I've had for many years that progressively got worse with age. I tried seeing two doctors, chiropractors, massages, and taking ibuprofen/mobic. My life was significantly interrupted due to this. I needed to cut out aerobics, weight training, and aggressive exercise, and cut work hours. After coming to The Back and Neck Relief Center, results were immediately apparent with improvement in comfort, range of motion, and function. I was able to also resume some exercise and dance. The staff are helpful in researching my insurance benefits to ensure that I can receive services. Very nice and attentive for a busy place!" - Barbara Phillips

*"Michael Greenspan's Neuromuscular Alignment System (NAS)
will become the gold standard in back and neck pain relief."*
Dr. Rand McClain

A Buddhist monk was walking along the shore with a disciple the morning after a terrible storm. There were several starfish trapped on the beach; they would certainly die if left out in the harsh sun. The monk bent down, picked one up and threw it back into the ocean. His disciple looked puzzled and asked him why he would do this when there were miles of beached starfish lying out in the sun. It can't possibly make a significant difference, he reasoned. The monk quietly picked up the next one and said to the disciple "It makes a difference to this one" and threw it into the ocean as well.

Do what you can for the people around you; it may not change the whole world, but it will change that one person's world.

This book was written on just that principle. It is my hope that through reading this book, you can come to a greater understanding of the human form as it relates to the muscular-skeletal system, more specifically back and neck pain, and that you are able to see the importance of high quality soft-tissue therapy work in the lives of yourself and others. If a neuromuscular alignment therapist helps just one person to be able to walk freely and comfortably again, then their job is done.

TABLE OF CONTENTS

INTRODUCTION

I played a lot of sports from a young age: basketball, soccer, baseball, gymnastics. I loved to play all types of sports, my favorite was basketball, it was like my church, my temple, my place of solace at a very young age, most likely the place I channeled all my energy growing up without a dad who died when I was 1 years old. I was very internally driven to compete and be the best I could, no male role model, just my mom and sister.

Then, I broke my back playing sports. It was an ongoing fracture or break in my lower back L5-S1 due to early childhood gymnastics and the constant pounding of basketball. One day I woke up with excruciating low back pain that seemed much worse, so my mom took me to the doctors. MRI and x-rays showed I had a broken vertebra.

I couldn't walk, my friends had to carry me off the basketball court one day, I suffered tons of pain, missed a third of my senior year of basketball, and so on. My mom brought me to all sorts of treatments, chiropractors, surgeons, physical therapists, massage therapists, and more. My mom was at the mercy of the medical community, she just didn't know what to do. I suffered with back pain for years, went to a ton of practitioners, all to no avail. I tried different types of Chiropractors and Massage Therapists. The Chiros cracked my bones and irritated the L5/S1 joint, shook it up like a hornet's nest, and re-inflamed it completely. The massages just felt like they were almost tickling the area with a feather and dancing around the pain, barely coming close to the source of it. Some physicians recommended back surgery, to fuse my vertebra, and I am so glad that I resisted that, as I finally got most of my first magical lasting relief a few years later with a neuromuscular massage instructor, and longer magical relief following the treatment protocol I outline later, beginning with a specific type of therapy to get rid of the spasms in the soft-tissues.

I attended college at The University of Colorado, Boulder, where I majored in Kinesiology/Exercise Physiology in order to begin my journey towards Medical School. However, like many collegians I was deflected from this goal because I fell in love. Yes, I fell in love with muscles and the muscular skeletal system because of my journey suffering from back pain. I soon learned that less than 3% of the medical school curriculum is devoted to the muscular-skeletal system, and it was my mission early on to truly help people get rid of pain for good through other evidence-based natural methods, rather than prescribing awful pain pills or having surgery. I wanted to help back pain sufferers just like I was, to heal and live a pain-free life like myself, and I knew unless I became a surgeon I wasn't going to be hands-on helping people get rid of pain. I knew surgery wasn't the path for me. I avoided it at all costs to eventually be pain-free in my back.

While a full-time student at University of Colorado in Boulder getting my college degree, I attended a second separate school for two years to learn elite manual therapy and soft-tissue therapy hands-on skills.

What did that entail? I was full-time at University Colorado, Boulder, then after class went an additional 20 hours + per week for two years at the same time, to a second school where I studied all types of manual therapy, soft-tissue training, and specialized in neuromuscular therapy for serious pain relief. After graduating from both schools in 1995, I moved to Telluride, Colorado for a year to live, work, and ski some more. I continued my hunger for more knowledge and became a seminar junkie, flying around the country taking as many seminars as possible from the most world-renowned experts in many types of modalities for serious pain relief. I integrated all my knowledge to create my own courses eventually and taught Neuromuscular Therapy to massage therapists, personal trainers, chiropractors, doctors and any health practitioners wanting more advanced soft-tissue and manual therapy skills.

It was at this time in 1994, while in college, that I opened up my first private practice office in Boulder, helping back and neck pain sufferers live pain-free lives. I utilized and tied together all the evidence-based treatments I learned that I still do today, from soft-tissue manual therapy, biomechanics, postural alignment corrective exercise therapy, dynamic stretching, and joint mobilizations.

Eventually, I began to teach and practice, and create my own method called NAS, Neuromuscular Alignment System.

More information about me or my activities can be found on our website at <ins>http://www.MassageRevolution.com</ins>

Here is what I have learned in my more than two decades of practice.

Many of the ideas about back and neck pain are simply wrong. This is, in part, because many in the medical profession have not been taught and therefore don't understand the real reasons behind this raging epidemic. In fact, the emphasis on merely treating the symptom, generally through medications and surgery, that characterizes the US health system *merely contributes to the problem*. In fact, nowhere is this emphasis on treating symptoms rather than causes shown to be more inadequate than in the treatment of back, neck and joint pain in general.

It is estimated that there are almost half a million spinal fusions conducted in the US every year; many of these aren't justified by what we know about the real causes of back pain. Moreover, even when they are 'successful', such surgeries don't address the cause. Sure, they can provide relief from the pain for a while, but without addressing the cause they might just be delaying the inevitable return of the pain and even disability. The fact is that the most successful treatments of back pain require neither surgery nor drugs. Let me say that again…

The fact is that the most successful treatments of back pain require neither surgery nor drugs.

In my clinics, the first thing we do is something you almost certainly won't get when you go to your doctor. Can you guess what it is?

Where would it make sense to focus an assessment?

Would it be to take a history of your pain relief attempts, i.e. medications?

Would it be to feel your spine?

Would it be to prescribe an MRI?

The first place we look and where we pay most attention is to where the *cause of the problem* lies.

We do a comprehensive assessment of your *posture, muscle balance, and knots in your back called 'trigger points'*. And armed with that information we set about healing your back pain without resorting to long-term medications or surgery.

The reasons for this approach, what you have to do to actually fix your back and neck pain, and the overwhelming evidence for its success, I reveal in the remaining pages of this book.

Are you tired of living with back or neck pain? When you have read this book you are armed with all the necessary information to heal your back, neck and joint problems without the need for expensive procedures that don't effectively address the problem. Good luck!!

***

CHAPTER ONE

WHO GETS LOW BACK AND NECK PAIN?

Low back pain is an often mistreated and potentially dangerous disorder that affects the lives of millions of Americans each year. It is one of humanity's most frequent complaints. It affects about 90% of Americans at some point in their lives and there are an estimated 480,000 yearly spinal fusion surgeries in the United States alone, and that number is rising. Between 2004-2008, an estimated 2.06 million episodes of lower back pain occurred in the US alone. Each year, low back pain accounts for 3.15% of all emergency visits with 65% of low back injuries occurring at home. It's the leading cause of job-related disability and missed work days, as five out of ten working adults have it every year.

Low back pain (LBP) is a widespread complaint in the United States. It is the fifth most common complaint for which professional health care advice is sought. Neck pain is similarly widespread. Studies suggest an annual prevalence of neck pain ranging between 30% and 50%, with one review reporting an average rate of 37.2%. The estimated lifetime prevalence of neck pain ranges from between 22% to 70%.

From 1994 to 2005, MRI scans of the lumbar region increased by more than 300% in Medicare beneficiaries.

37% of Americans who experience low back pain don't seek professional help.

The majority of people (8 out of 10) initially seek help from their primary care physician or a chiropractor. The remaining 2 out of 10 see a subspecialist for treatment.

In the US, two to five percent of all doctor's visits are for back pain, which equals:

$86 billion in healthcare costs.

While it is estimated that 80% of Americans experience low back pain during their lifetime, surveys suggest that at any one time that number is between 30-35%. That's a lot of people, especially when you add in similar numbers for neck pain!

According to recent research, more than 25% of adults have had a *recent* episode of low back pain. Women tend to have greater prevalence than men, older people have a greater prevalence than younger ones, and long hours and work satisfaction are related to the condition. It is estimated that low back pain costs the country more than $100 billion annually when factoring in all the related costs.

Low back pain occurs all over the world, although the incidence varies which sheds some light on the real basis of the problem. Worldwide, low back pain is the single greatest cause of disability, and ranks sixth in terms of "overall disease burden". Those of European or African ancestry have significantly higher rates of lower back pain when compared with those of Asian ancestry. Chronic low back pain has a profound socioeconomic impact on individuals, families, and communities – so much that the World Health Organization has identified it as a major disabling condition.

Despite this onslaught of sad statistics, the good news is that you do not have to suffer. Neither do your family members, neighbors, friends or colleagues. If you don't suffer from back or neck pain I'm sure you know several people who do. When you have finished reading the book, you're able to spread the word and help heal your loved ones. And if you do suffer from back or neck pain, the relief you get from my cure will enhance all your relationships. Pain is stressful and it affects the entire family.

If you do suffer from back and neck pain I am sure you have frequently wondered about it, if not obsessed about it.
Questions like...

- Why does my back hurt so much?
- Why doesn't the pain ever go away?
- Why can't I just be normal?

- Will I eventually be unable to move at all?

- What will life look like in five, ten, fifteen years?

This book helps you answer those questions and shows those concerns, while understandable, it is easily and successfully resolved. You get the answers to those questions in the following pages and you are able to find relief and hope.

The fact is that back pain does impact the quality of your life.

Unfortunately, telling people about the unseen problems caused by back pain only makes them feel more frustrated – at first. They can see it can be as debilitating as they often feel. But then they learn the way to eliminate the back pain and they then can truly appreciate what a gift that cure is. As a young man, I experienced that frustration and hopelessness. I had all that energy, all those dreams and I was concerned I would never be able to realize them. Perhaps for me that was the hardest part of my journey – the fear that my back problems would rob me of life. You might be feeling that, too. Don't worry – just read on.

Moreover, back pain severely restricts movement and it turns out that movement is key not just to physical health but brain health, too. In fact, the reduction in movement is one of the biggest factors in "aging." Those who maintain their freedom and range of movement don't "age" like others and keep their lives and mental and physical faculties going full on into their eighties and nineties.

Movement is essential for physical and mental well-being. We now know the detrimental effects of being sedentary. They're not just physical, like an increase of heart disease, stroke, obesity, diabetes, and even dementia. Lack of movement impacts how your mind and brain function. For example, during movement, important chemicals are released that are crucial for a healthy brain, like Brain-Derived Neurotropic Factor (BDNF) which is like "Miracle Gro" for brain cells. And we have learnt in the past decade or so, that the brain can continually grow new brain cells and brain pathways that are the key to functioning well as we age. In fact, the biggest contributor to the development of new brain cells through the lifespan is – exercise and movement. Back pain isn't just a problem in your back. If movement is rendered difficult through back or neck pain – or frankly anything – the impact is wide-reaching. As you soon learn, there are trigger points that immobilize you and without fixing them, your back is in pain, your movement restricted, and you suffer mentally as well as physically.

I know that you have probably tried to "suck it up" or ignore the pain. However, hoping it might go away someday is not a treatment. As the saying goes, "Someday is not a day of the week". In fact, ignoring the pain only makes it worse over time. Back pain has a tendency to get worse without the right attention. While there might be periods of temporary relief, it is likely to get worse over time. The fact is that you have an underlying problem that is not getting treated and only gets worse. As you read in the following pages, you're making it worse every day by trying to compensate for it.

You might not know how it started but that doesn't matter. The only thing that you need to know is the nature of the problem and the cure.

So, what are your choices?

I'm sure you have already tried prescription and even non-prescription medications, possibly surgery, or other treatments, but the problem is always there.

Let me share with you the story of a woman named Pattie.

Pattie is a 44-year old mother of two who works in the HR department of a local corporation. Pattie has suffered from an occasional mild low back pain but because it usually goes away after a couple of days, she didn't pay it much attention.

One day, as she was leaning over to feed the copier machine, she felt the pain in her back. Except this was much more intense than it had ever been. She struggled gamely through the rest of her day and couldn't wait to get home and lay down.

When her husband came home, he checked out her spine. He is a doctor and suggested that if she stay off her feet for a while, the pain would likely subside. He did give her a pain reliever.

After an hour or so, Pattie did begin to feel better. She reassured herself she would be able to go to work the next day and be OK. She was taking pain relievers every four hours and wanted to wean herself off them. However, the pain returned pretty quickly, so she decided that she just needed the medication to keep her going.

There's something important to know about pain relievers. They don't actually get rid of the pain. They mask it by disabling your brain's ability to feel pain. Interestingly, placebo pills (dummy pills) work the same way.

So, the pain hasn't gone anywhere, your brain has been numbed. You may think that this is a technical point, and you don't care how the relief is achieved as long as the pain is gone. However, there is something critical to know here.

Pain is a warning sign that something is wrong. It is like a fire alarm, alerting you to trouble. The problem with pain meds is that they have turned off the fire alarm not put out the fire! You are still getting pain, your body is in big trouble, but you don't know it. In fact, it is getting worse even as you are feeling thankful that the pain has gone.

Not only that, because you have been numbed you don't realize that you are making the pain worse!!

Not only do painkillers risk making your condition worse, they also have unpleasant side-effects that develop, especially with continued use. Common over-the-counter painkillers can cause stomach, kidney, liver and brain issues. Prescription drugs, especially opioids, are very addictive and often difficult to withdraw from.

After three months of regularly taking pain meds, Pattie realized she was not getting any better. To make matters worse, she was growing increasingly stressed and irritable at home and work. Everyone was feeling it. Her husband, the family doctor and the doctor in the family, tried all the things he had been taught in medical school, but these were all variations of medication cocktails. Pattie and her husband both knew that it was a bad idea for him to try to treat her, so he referred his wife to a physician who had known Pattie since she was a teenager. Surely, he would know how to solve this situation?

After reminiscing for a few minutes, Pattie and Dr. Johnson talked about the problem she had come to see him about. Dr. Johnson surmised that Pattie had strained a few muscles as a result of her work and he noted that she had not taken any time off for her back to recover. He smiled as he wrote out a prescription for a new medication cocktail of pain and stress relievers. He emphasized that

she should stay in bed and not do anything for a few days and that
she would soon be able to put the back pain behind her.

Pattie did exactly as Dr. Johnson had said. She slept a lot, snuggled
with her kids and felt out of it most of the time. At the suggestion of
her husband, she stopped the meds on the third day and tried to get
up and move. But she was very stiff and before the evening was out,
felt her pain return. She cried inconsolably as her husband held her
helplessly in his arms.

Her husband was as frustrated as Pattie was. Here he was, a trained
doctor with years of practice and a great reputation but he just
didn't know how to help his own wife with back pain. He started to
wonder about some of the patients he had seen for the similar
condition. He had assumed that many of them had not come back to
him because they were cured. Now the realization struck him that
they might not have come back to him because they knew he couldn't
help them. He started to question what he did know about back pain
and the usual medical practice advice. He started to feel that he was
unqualified to treat the problem.

Pattie's husband realized first hand that most physicians are not
trained in how to really detect back pain and its causes. That's not
their area of expertise. Without the right expertise, they simply use
the standard conventional treatments for pain that at best numb the
pain for a while.

But here's what doctors need to know.

The significant causes of back and neck pain are muscle imbalances, trigger points, and tight or weak muscles which pull your body out of alignment. Even one slightly misaligned muscle can lead to a cascade of painful adaptations that can create severe pain. Treating only the pain does nothing about the underlying misalignment and weakness and the true cause of the pain remains.

You can only fix the problem by addressing these *trigger points,* imbalances and weaknesses. Pattie didn't understand this and neither did her husband. However, you now know the secret and if you follow the advice in the remaining pages you won't have to suffer like she did.

Patti and her husband called Dr. Johnson to see what more he could suggest as the prescribed medication and rest hadn't worked. Her husband's authority as a doctor seemed to give Dr. Johnson some pause, especially as both Pattie and her husband were concerned about her moods and the effect that all this was having on her children. She did yoga weekly and had always been very active with them and felt terrible that she could do nothing except read to them. Eventually, Dr. Johnson suggested that Pattie should try physical therapy. He referred her to a therapist who had an office in his building and reassured her that she would be soon back to normal.

Despite the fact that Pattie ached for a normal back as soon as possible, she wasn't convinced it was going to happen any time soon.

Traditional physical therapy can be sometimes helpful in dealing with back and neck pain. I sometimes send my own clients for such help.

Sometimes, however, it doesn't work and that can happen because the underlying problem has not been properly diagnosed. If your physician misdiagnoses the problem, his instructions to any health practitioner, including physical therapists, won't be helpful and hinder their effectiveness.

There can also be another problem with physical therapy. Many physical therapists emphasize strengthening exercises for out of balance muscles way too soon. While rehabbing injured soft-tissues and painful muscles, it's vital to stick with the principle of *"lengthen before you strengthen."* This is a part of my secret recipe for success I discuss later in the book.

Two months later, Pattie returned to her doctor. She was depressed and her life bore little resemblance to what it had just a few short months before. She had been unable to work, play with her kids, or pretty much do anything. The pain had gotten worse, spread to her neck and upper back, to the point where it was excruciating just to try to sit in a chair.

Dr. Johnson's expression said it all. He no longer had that hopeful smile and confident demeanor.

"Pattie, there's nothing more that I can do for you. I'm going to refer you to a local surgeon who I know. He's the best around here and seems to have some success."

Unfortunately, this scenario occurs daily in this country, and other countries, too. Surgery is a risky procedure especially if the diagnosis is less than 1000% accurate. In fact, research suggests that many people with chronic back problems show no physical abnormality on an MRI, and that people who report no back issues, have MRIs that show spinal abnormalities. Go figure. But be very wary before you Go Surgery.

Spinal surgery is often reported as one of the most ineffective surgical interventions with some research reporting a success rate of 47-50%. Moreover, some of those "successful" surgeries only bring short-term relief.

You do not have to live with your back or neck pain. There are other options apart from drugging yourself or consenting to have someone cut you open. You don't have to live with pain, numbness and immobility. You can have the life you want. There is a much better alternative! And fortunately for Pattie and you, I'm about to show you what it is.

It is being increasingly recognized by world leading authorities that trigger points, or small "landmine knots" in the back and neck muscles, are the main cause of more than 80% of cases of chronic back and neck pain. These trigger points are found in almost every back and neck pain sufferer. The best back pain relief experts are those who are very skilled in releasing these trigger points hands-on, using neuromuscular massage and trigger point therapy.

Unlike the typical medical treatments, this method doesn't sweep the problem under the rug, it addresses the problem -- and gives you a new rug and floors, too! And unlike conventional medical treatments, this methodology utilizes the body's natural healing process to untangle the problem.

Welcome back to your natural body and a life without pain. Goodbye medications, physician visits, and costly deductibles!

As a Neuromuscular Therapist, and owner of The Back and Neck Relief Center in Manhattan Beach, California, our Back & Neck Pain Relief Specialists are trained in evidence-based treatments for the detection and treatment of trigger points, muscle imbalances, and postural misalignments to restore natural form and ideally keep you permanently pain free.

Please don't fall into the trap of thinking that because we don't use medications and surgery, that we are low tech or old-fashioned. On the contrary, what I share with you in the rest of this book is very scientifically advanced, natural and, if you pardon the pun, cutting edge -- without any cuts. And it dramatically improves the quality of your life.

I've been treating people with back and neck pain for more than 27 years and I have seen first-hand how these techniques work.

As you learned in the introduction, I am totally dedicated to changing the lives of low back and neck pain sufferers by offering evidence-based, scientifically proven and advanced methods like neuromuscular therapy. This is my calling and my purpose. (Check out our testimonial sheet to hear what clients have to say about working with us!)

The chances are pretty high that we have treated people with the same problem you are suffering from right now. My colleagues and I understand exactly how you feel. You may recall that one of the main reasons I decided to become a neuromuscular alignment therapist was my own experience with horrendous back pain and no other therapies worked for me until I consulted with a neuromuscular therapist, who accurately diagnosed my problem and knew how to fix it.

My colleagues and I know that you're not imagining the pain. We know that it is all too real. Neither do we want you to simply get used to it. I know how helpless, frustrated and angry one can feel when life is restricted. I know how tough it is to tell your kids that you can't play with them right now, you just have to lie down and rest.

When you tell us your problems we're going to believe you, even if the radiologist can't see them on the X-ray.

We're never going to tell you that "there's nothing we can do," or that "you have to live with it."

Several university studies have declared the treatment I am about to describe in this book – Neuromuscular Alignment System -- as the *safest, most effective and all-natural evidence-based successful treatment of low back and neck pain.*

A few days before her surgery, Pattie's husband saw an old patient of his in his clinic. The patient told him that the meds that he had prescribed for his back pain really didn't work but he had finally found something that did. He described how he had come to our clinic and was fully assessed and treated with our unique neuromuscular alignment system. The patient looked like a totally different man. The doctor was thrilled, not just for the old man. He immediately called Pattie and told her the news.

Pattie came to our clinic the next day, explaining that her husband had just seen the results of our treatment on one of his old patients. Could this work for her?

I sat down with Pattie and listened to her story. I then explained in some detail the same method I'm writing about in this book

Pattie's reaction was typical. Her whole face lit up and she almost pleaded with me to do an assessment right away. Following a brief posture, muscle balance, and trigger point assessment, I noticed a couple of problem areas that were likely the cause of the problem. We created a program to get her life back. A life without pain, frustration, anger, meds or surgery.

Pattie now has her life back. She's reports being pain-free and feeling awesome!

It's really cool to see our clients make such wonderful recoveries. While I can't boast about having the ability to treat every condition that every person can suffer from, I do feel honored to be considered one of the leading authorities in the treatment of back and neck pain in all of Los Angeles!

I encourage you to not just read this book but also *to take action*. The easiest way to deal with any problem is to minimize it, pretend it isn't that bad, or deny it exists at all. That's simply the path to even more pain. Get it fixed! After reading this book you see that it is not only possible but easier than you think.

Today, healthcare has become more complex as a function of how much more we know about different conditions, their causes and treatments. So, in any aspect of your health it is key to work with the experts in your problem. As we have seen, the typical internist is a jack-of-all trades, who might not understand about the subtleties of your back, neck and other muscular pains. Having some experience in prescribing medications or surgery is nowhere near sufficient expertise for actually assessing and treating what underlies most back problems. Seek advice and help from people like me, who have made getting rid of low back and neck pain their life's purpose.

Now that you have learned who has the answers to your back problems, don't stop now. Read the remaining pages to get more insight into the treatment you need. And don't forget that the difference between those who are liberated from their back and neck pain and those who live in misery is that the former seek out the real experts and take action.

***

CHAPTER TWO

WHY BACK AND NECK PAIN ARE SO COMMON

We're not born to have poor posture. We're actually born with a healthy postural blueprint, yet over time muscle imbalances assaulted by the force of gravity start having their way with our posture and structure.

Basically, the gist for Why is Back/Neck Pain So Common is….

- Babies are born with a perfect "design" for health and function.
- We grow up in a society that lacks movement (we go from bed to the car to the desk/computer to the coach/TV to the bed and then repeat the entire cycle).
- We grow up in a society that lacks functional movement. Our ancestors did a lot more manual work, and healthier functional movements, movements that our muscles and joints actually must have and need in order to remain functionally healthy. They squatted down low a lot or lunged, which is essential for healthy muscle balance and function of your hips, pelvis, core, and back, and puts the hip joint through its full range of motion. Today, people rarely squat, hence it deprives your hip and back muscles/joints to go through their full range of healthy motion, hence the high

number of hip replacements and back pain in our culture. This leads to muscle imbalance and dysfunction.

- Our ancestors also lifted things more, especially overhead, which is essential for healthy muscle balance and function of the shoulders and upper back. Today, people work at computers and hold their TV remote, and they hardly ever do activities overhead, like reaching overhead, which deprives their shoulders and backs of the full range of motion and healthy muscle balance and function, which leads to back/neck pain.

- Lack of healthy muscle balance and function leads to poor posture, postural distortions, which then leads to trigger points, which then creates the back/neck pain. This is key!

- There are rarely practitioners with advanced hands-on palpation skills capable of getting to and eliminating these pain-creating trigger point sources.

- Even when a highly skilled practitioner gets rid of the pain-creating trigger point sources, and relieves the pain, in order to cure it and permanently end the pain, it's vital that the back/neck pain sufferer then gets even further to the root cause of their pain by fixing all their muscle imbalances and dysfunctions.

Whoever suggested that it might be an adaptive advantage for humans to stand on two legs didn't provide the appropriate caveat: Two legs are cool and has lots of advantages *if you stand up straight with healthy muscle balance and alignment.*

The evidence suggests that for several thousand years, humans did a good job of standing erect. Then industrialization and more recently technology, changed human's stature – and posture.

If you look at some of the earliest videos that go back more than a century, one thing is striking especially in movies of Americans. One of my favorites is a movie shot around 1910 in New York. On the streets of Manhattan, you see both men and women dressed in what today we would consider formal attire. There are women with parasols and long dresses, men in suits and top hats. These clothes were a reflection of, and contribution to, the culture, a culture in which standing upright was the norm. Have you ever seen a guy with a slumped posture walking along wearing a top hat? No, because if you're slumped the damned hat would keep falling off! What is also noticeable in those early movies is that the vast majority of people look positively anorexic compared to today's population.

The rise of convenience has not only meant less physical movement and activity, which in itself has disastrous health consequences, but also led to significant changes in posture, especially in western and first world countries.

34

In an extreme example, if you live in a first world country, you simply get water by going to the faucet and turning it on, or even going to the pantry or refrigerator and get water that is already bottled for you. However, in other parts of the world, you are not so "lucky." You have to walk a few miles to water sources, fill up as many stone vessels as you can carry, and walk home balancing at least one of the full pots on your head. The effort involved might be a proverbial pain in the you-know-what, but it does offer extreme protection against real back and neck pain. In first world countries it seems absurd to be able to carry full water pots on your head while walking – the total opposite of what we expect or want to do. However, the price paid for this false perception is back and neck pain, endless medications and numerous surgeries.

In short, we don't engage in movements that specifically keep our posture upright and our bodies in alignment. In the modern world, we don't have to and while that may seem a blessing, the curse comes in the form of severe back and neck pain.

The massive change from physical labor to sedentary work also has compounded the problem. In sedentary positions, especially in today's culture, your head drops forward, leading to a slouched position. So, if you're working at the computer, chances are good that your device is not at eye level, but considerably lower, resulting in a slouch.

Fact: For every inch of forward head posture, it's 10lbs of gravitational force compressing your neck muscles and vertebra

Solution: When sitting at the computer, keep your head over your shoulders, avoid "poking" your head forward. Looking from side, you want your ear directly over your shoulders! (see Figure A)

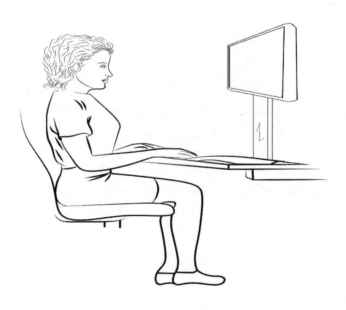

Figure A: Good sitting posture alignment

The other day I was in a certain well-known coffee location and there was a woman, sitting on a stool reading a book. She looked out of place and a little odd because rather than having the book in her lap, she was holding it up with her hands at eye level thus maintaining an upright posture (see Figure A). Yes, even in our leisure activities, especially in our leisure activities, we slump and slouch. One benefit of the advent of wall-mounted televisions is that they are typically mounted higher than free standing TVs and thus require us to hold our heads up rather than slouch. But then your sitting posture can get you into serious trouble (see Figure B)

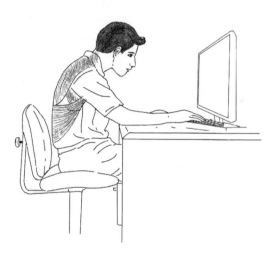

Figure B: Bad sitting posture alignment

The slumped posture becomes even more problematic and out of alignment when we add weight like groceries, backpacks and young children. When you are out of alignment extra weight only compounds the muscular imbalances leading to more pain creating trigger points and even more dysfunction.

With all of these differences, some of which have been enhanced by fashion trends, it's hardly surprising that back and neck pain have become increasingly problematic (and top hats are now out of vogue.)

These trends have also contributed to the reciprocal relationship between obesity and back and neck pain. The more back and neck pain, the less likelihood of healthy movement, leading to a reduced caloric need, leading to excess weight, leading to more back and neck pain in a very painful cycle. Back and neck pain also influences other lifestyle behaviors, like sleep, which are critical to health. Poor sleep is associated with both increased weight as well as increased risk of cardiovascular disease and overall morbidity.

On the critical subject of sleep, healthy sleep (defined as 7 to 8 hours of restorative sleep) relaxes muscles more, and healthier muscles function better to keep you pain-free, with less toxin buildup, better circulation, fewer pain-creating trigger points!

Moreover, poor sleep, which nearly half the population reports, is associated with accidents of all sorts, from falls to car crashes, that can seriously impact your musculature. More about that shortly.

The human body has evolved to support its weight through the skeleton and with the use of muscles. While this seems obvious, if you are reading this from the United States, the chances are that your muscles are chronically doing extra work to support your body.

Differentiate the following postures: Figures C and D show good muscle balance and function, naturally aligning their spine, pelvic center, knees and ankles, as if on a plumb line, with their structural alignment supporting their weight while Figures E and F slump their shoulders and back and crane their neck. Who will experience back pain? Figures E and F.

Figure C: Good Standing Posture Alignment

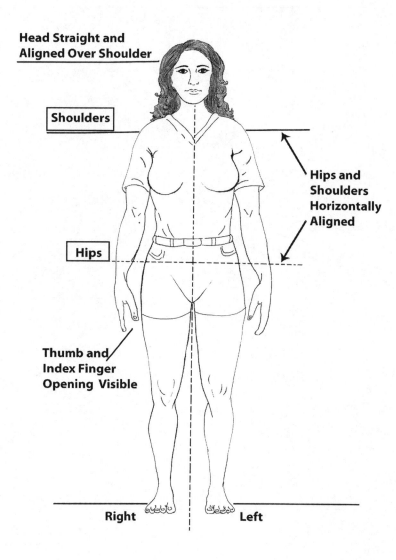

Head Straight and Aligned Over Shoulder

Shoulders

Hips and Shoulders Horizontally Aligned

Hips

Thumb and Index Finger Opening Visible

Right   **Left**

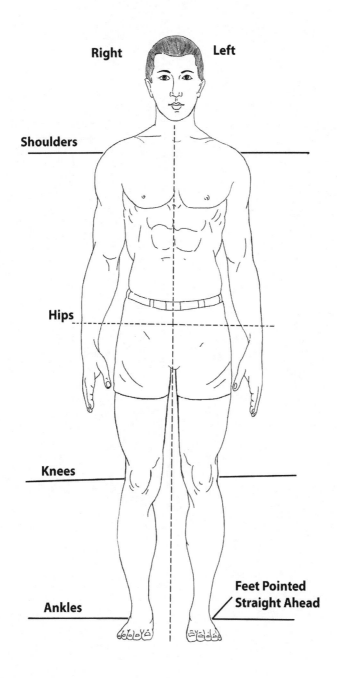

Figure D: Good Standing Posture Alignment

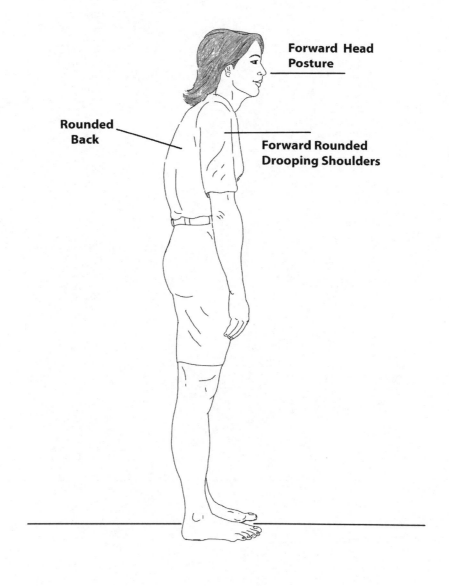

Forward Head Posture

Rounded Back

Forward Rounded Drooping Shoulders

Figure E: Poor Standing Posture Alignment

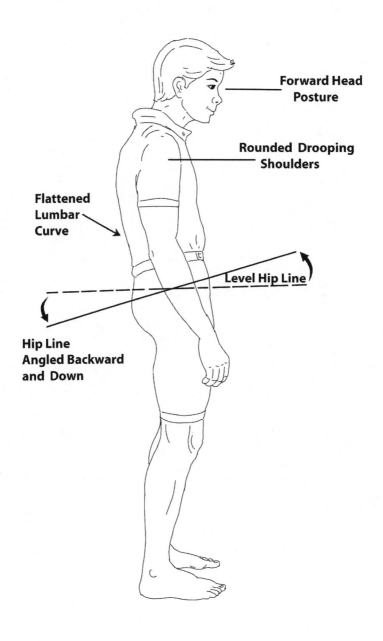

Forward Head Posture

Rounded Drooping Shoulders

Flattened Lumbar Curve

Level Hip Line

Hip Line Angled Backward and Down

Figure F: Poor Standing Posture Alignment

Unfortunately, most Americans are likely to identify more with figures E and F. The slumped posture, shoulders bent, eyes (and therefore head) facing down pulling the neck forward. And we're not just, or even, talking about seniors – this applies to the young and old.

If Americans were more vigilant about their muscle balance, function, posture and ensured a more upright stance and conveyed this to their children, many back, neck, knee and muscular problems in all generations could be avoided.

The difference between healthy and unhealthy posture can be clearly seen when looking at people in places like Portugal and Bali, where back and neck pain is uncommon. A French researcher, Noelle Perez, showed that in these countries the natural standing posture is much more erect. When these populations do suffer from muscular problems they are more likely to derive from poor nutrition and accidents, but common activities like sitting, carrying children, or bending do not produce pain.

***

CHAPTER THREE

WESTERN SOCIETY HAS LOST ITS FUNCTION

Okay, so we have become more sedentary, but why is that really a problem apart from lack of movement?

The problem is that when muscles aren't used they effectively shut down. Without activity and good blood flow, muscles go to sleep. The connections with the brain go quiet, which isn't good for structures that are designed to be active. The only way to activate them is to move. Without such activity, muscles will atrophy causing the imbalances and trigger points that underpin almost all back and neck pain.

Modern life and the drive for convenience hasn't just changed our posture, it has changed our movement.

We sleep in customized ultra-comfortable beds, travel in a sedentary position, sit all day in a chair staring down at the computer, and relax on very accommodating couches. As I mentioned earlier, we barely ever squat or reach overhead anymore to activate the full range of motion of our hip and shoulder muscles!

So, we've created a society with unused and pissed off muscles, which retaliate by causing muscular knots and trigger points and the back and neck pain that ensue. It's almost as if your muscles are saying, "You don't want to use me, then I'll show you what that is really going to feel like!"

If you're kinder to your muscles and do get to move during the day and make them feel worthwhile, they can relent. Even muscles need self-confidence.

You may be familiar with the famous children's story "The Little Engine That Could". Everyone doubted that the little engine could actually support a heavy load and pull it successfully to its destination.

Then there is The Little Muscle That Could: Could help coordinate movement, persist and show its strength and resilience. We need to empower our muscles so they turn "I think I can, I think I can," into "Of course, I can." Don't give your muscles self-esteem problems by not using them and trusting them.

In the case of *eventual movement*, rather than effectively no movement, the muscles relent, they don't get so uptight and the pain can begin to diminish. This is why for some people the pain can be varying or even intermittent. However, that is also misleading as it can lead many people to underestimate the potential long-term impact of muscular imbalance and trigger points. It also leads them to accept a degree of discomfort and restriction, which not only is unacceptable but also unnecessary.

So, we're losing function as a "sitting" culture where we use and keep creating all sorts of things to "accommodate" us, supposedly make our lives easier, yet they're diminishing the sole purpose, design, function of the human body, which is to move.

I used to say that "Bill Gates built my practice," producing a never ending supply of back/neck pain sufferers at the computer, as the computer and computer worker have become a catalyst for the onslaught of the back pain sufferers. Muscles shut down when you sit, they turn to jelly, mush, the neurological "lights" turn off like when you shut off your lights in your house and it goes dark. If your muscles could scream out they'd be saying "Hey, who turned off the lights, it's dark in here, and feels like a prison!"

The only way to save them and turn the light switch back "on" is to get up and move! To do that though, you often first need to get out of the pain, which is where getting advanced bodywork and muscle relief work comes in to play, especially releasing the pain causing "landmine knots" known as trigger points.

We've advanced further than ever as a society, living longer, yet are we healthier? In just the last 50 years there's been a huge decline as a society in healthy functional movement, and "a muscle that gets no play will waste away." Muscles have minds of their own; they need movement, blood flow, stretching, activation, play and motion.

Otherwise muscles form pain causing trigger points inside them and bite you back with pain.

Now we've got a society with "upset" muscles, which lash out at you by causing the painful landmine knots better known as trigger points. With a fiery vengeance, these trigger points in your muscles rear their ugly head causing you to suffer from back pain, neck pain, and more, until someone with the "all-mighty" thumb comes by to help you and de-activate them. The most effective way to release, relieve, and de-activate painful trigger points is with manual direct pressure - there's no way around it.

The current state of western society also creates incredible demands that lead to feeling overwhelmed and stressed, which is bad for your body.

Sleep and Back Pain

One of the problems of the western world is lack of sleep. The body (and brain) need a good balance of stimulation and rest. For many people today, there is a massive imbalance between being "on" and taking time to adequately restore themselves. For example, the recommendation is that the ideal amount of sleep per night is between 7 and 8 hours. Many people in the US, perhaps at least half, don't get adequate sleep, and about 35% have diagnosable sleep disorders like insomnia, and sleep apnea. Many people claim they only need 5 or 6 hours a night but that are likely to be wrong. They might be able to get by on less than 7 hours a night, but they would function much better on 7-8; they just don't know it. Poor sleep is likely to affect you in several ways that exacerbate back and neck problems. The more tired you are, the more you are likely to stoop, sit for long periods, and be generally less active.

Lack of sleep is also a major contributor to accidents of all types, less than optimal performance in all areas, increased risk of disease, and even relationship issues.

5% of people actually admit to driving in a drowsy state or actually falling asleep at the wheel, which can lead to accidents that results in serious back, neck and other problems.

Poor sleep is also highly related to obesity and cardiovascular disease. The stress, immune and hormone systems are all affected by poor sleep. Poor sleep is also associated with a higher risk of cognitive decline and dementia, especially because recent research shows that one of the main functions of sleep is clearing toxins from the brain. Toxins like tau and amyloid, which are both highly implicated in Alzheimer's Disease.

Poor sleep will also affect your ability to reduce inflammation and tolerate pain.

Emotional and physical fatigue that are the result of poor sleep are also likely to contribute to poor posture, a lot more sitting and less physical activity, which can create back and neck pain in the first place, as well as make it much difficult to manage and tolerate once it has developed.

Sleeping position is also critical to retaining good muscle balance, healthy muscles, and pain-free back and neck.

Figure G: Sleeping on one's back

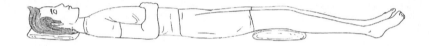

Sleeping on your back with a very thin pillow under your neck and knees is ideal (Figure G), as your body is in the best muscle balanced, postural aligned position.

If you must sleep on your side, to keep your body aligned as possible, use a pillow under your top arm and between your knees (Figure H).

The worst position for your neck, back, and pelvis is on your stomach (Figure I).

Figure H; Side-sleeping

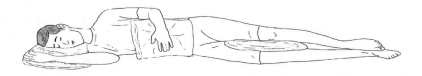

Figure I: Stomach sleeping

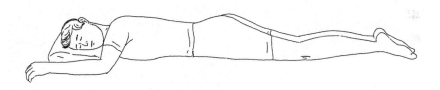

Nutrition

The Standard American Diet (SAD) can also contribute to muscular problems and pain. Poor nutrition also contributes to back and neck pain by adding excess weight. A high intake of sugar, for example, drinking several sodas a day, likely increases inflammation, as well as ultimately adds to fatigue. The Standard American Diet is also high in sugar and dairy, both of which contribute to weight gain and. inflammation

Exercise

A sedentary lifestyle also contributes to poor physical health as well as back and neck pain. We are made to move, and lack of adequate exercise is going to potentially contribute to joint pain and other problems. Lack of exercise also decreases energy, inhibits immune function and renders one less capable of the emotional resilience needed to deal with such problems. And some recent research suggests that upper and lower muscle strength are associated with cognitive function. Typically, handgrip is the simple measure used to assess muscle strength, but it shows little correlation to cognitive performance whereas upper and lower body muscle strength do show such an association.

Emotion Management

There are many levels that affect and cause your back pain, neck pain, and more pain. The majority of this book discusses the physical causes and solutions, yet in order to provide you the most thorough all-comprehensive pain healing guide, it's crucial to give you the complete recipe to cure your pain. Which means touching upon one all-important factor to back and neck pain, which is the emotional component.

HEALING IS APPLYING LOVE TO THE PLACES INSIDE THAT HURT

Inner anger, resentments, and rage so often manifest themselves in your physical body as physical pain, low back pain, upper back pain, neck pain, shoulder pain, and more, not to mention the even worse consequences of disease. Energetically within your body, anger has a "burning" affect upon your soft-tissues, like a fire inferno of hell, in your muscles, tendons, fascia, etc., which you may experience physically as pain. People come to our clinic, The Back & Neck Relief Center, seeking pain relief from symptoms being physically manifested as deeper core trauma issues. You can get all the treatments in the world yet the bottom line is you still must deal with these core issues that may be constantly fueling the pain body. Kill the fuel source and you've got true inner healing.

Dr. John Sarno is well-known for his belief that all back pain is emotionally charged and caused by anger. For me that's an overstatement because I see how trigger points and landmine knots occur as a result of poor posture not just, or even, poor emotional regulation. However, there is no question, that your emotional state influences your body, increasing pain and the risks of inflammation and soft tissue problems. Moreover, emotions affect body posture, thus creating trigger points and landmine knots. For example, consider the posture associated with sadness, depression and grief. Do those moods suggest an upright posture or a sagging, misaligned demeanor? Unfortunately, we live in a world where emotionalism is encouraged and is mischaracterized as 'authenticity', 'passion' or 'masculinity'. It also leads to pain and functional problems.

In short, the western lifestyle facilitates back, neck and other aches and pains by embracing more muscle imbalance and physically dysfunctional behaviors. Being healthy has to be, therefore, a very conscious choice to run counter to the natural tendencies implicit in the culture.

***

CHAPTER FOUR

5 COMMON MYTHS ABOUT TREATMENT

I have already referenced the research that suggests that many people without back pain also show bulging disks on an MRI. Is this an indictment of the reliability of the MRI? Well, these imaging machines do need to be calibrated correctly as evidenced by one piece of research that showed that dead salmon had positive brain imaging responses when shown pictures of humans. However, these variations in imaging are more likely to reflect how dynamic and remarkable the body's natural healing abilities are. You can see a structural malfunction one day but not another as the body quickly compensates.

Unfortunately, however, Western medicine is not typically based on a holistic view and focuses mainly on treating symptoms not underlying causes, especially where significant pain is involved. Again, it's all about convenience and speed rather than real efficacy. This leads to an emphasis on surgery and drugs, rather than addressing the causes. And these "remedies" not only can be ineffective as far as the main problem is concerned, they can create other problems, too, like severe and potentially damaging drug side-effects.

Eastern culture works cooperatively with nature, western culture works competitively with it, seeking to dominate and alter it. Additionally, western culture overvalues independence whereas eastern culture values interdependence. The cultural philosophies are fundamentally different, and therefore so are their treatment approaches. So, it's not that eastern approaches have been around longer, or are more mystical, it is that they are focused on addressing the problem from a holistic, cooperative perspective.

These philosophical differences lead to some important myths, that can seriously mislead the uninformed and even the informed person.

MYTHS

MYTH #1: ALL TYPES OF TREATMENTS ARE CREATED EQUAL

There are many great practitioners and different types of treatments in the various sectors of the health field. In my area of expertise, many of these "experts" proclaim themselves as "back and neck pain experts". And, for sure, many can often give you some relief. Temporary relief is not a permanent solution, though. I am assuming you want the latter, a permanent solution that addresses the causes not temporary relief that just gives you, well. …temporary relief.

The secret to the cure comes when using the body's natural resources to more effectively adapt, what I call Neuromuscular Alignment System or NAS.

If you think about the concept of adaptation, any adaptation, the sequence is important. So, for example, if you needed to adapt against a possible threat, the first step is ensuring you can identify the threat, devising a strategy to deal with the threat and so on. You wouldn't effectively start with planning what to do after you have defeated or encountered the threat. Your plan would be out of sequence.

Similarly, with the adaptation within the body, especially with adaptation and alignment of the body's natural resources, sequence is an essential part of the equation. So, in healing and rehabilitating injured muscles, *the sequence and order of therapy is CRITICAL.*

When you have back and neck pain, you have spasms, hyper-constrictions, and trigger points in your soft-tissues. Reason suggests, therefore, that first thing you MUST do *is end these spasms.*

Sure, you could have a chiropractor crack your bones, an acupuncturist treat you like a quilt and put needles all over your body, and have your doctor prescribe pain pills. Worst yet, you can have a physical therapist or trainer start strengthening exercises way too soon and before the spasms have been relieved.

The first, and only, place to start is having a highly skilled bodyworker release these soft-tissue spasms. It's the natural first stop in the adaptation process.

The unfortunate truth is that these awful muscle spasms, constrictions, landmine knots and trigger points don't just disappear when someone cracks your bones or sticks needles in you, or when you take a powerful narcotic. They also don't miraculously disappear when someone gives you strengthening exercises. As a result of these considerations, back and neck pain sufferers are often sold a bill of goods, because the trigger point knots at the source of the pain remain.

If you go for weekly bone adjustments when your muscles are tight, those trigger points and muscle imbalances are just going to pull them right back to where they were again. You'll be enhancing your chiropractor's practice and retirement plan with a treatment regimen that doesn't work. You are out of alignment in both your muscles and your adaptation strategy.

MYTH #2: YOU CAN STRETCH YOUR WAY OUT OF PAIN

Financially, your treatment might be a stretch, but the initial treatment itself shouldn't involve stretching.

If one could stretch oneself out of back, neck and other muscular pain, the pharmaceutical industry would be in trouble.

YOU CAN'T STRETCH YOUR WAY OUT OF MUSCULAR PAIN.

As I have pointed out, it's the muscle imbalances and trigger points that keep your muscles tight and in pain, making it very difficult to stretch. And just stretching won't get rid of the trigger points. The secret to reducing and eventually eliminating trigger points is DIRECT hands-on pressure. That hands-on work has to occur first and if it doesn't, those knots remain, creating pain and discomfort no matter how much stretching you do.

Additionally, overactive muscle tone, which is a characteristic of muscle spasm, creates 'hypertonic' muscle fibers.

Strengthening exercises and trying to strengthen hypertonic muscles merely over-activates them, making the pain and the problem worse.

That's why it is crucial to remove the muscle spasm first, lengthening the overly hypertonic muscle fibers. As we say it is critical to "Lengthen Before You Strengthen!" This is done with expert hands-on massage and bodywork, using direct manual pressure on the muscle and trigger point to release it, as well as using tools like foam rollers for self-treatment of trigger points in the muscles.

IMPORTANT: *Lengthen BEFORE You Strengthen!*

MYTH #3: YOU THROW OUT YOUR BACK.

Do you really "throw your back out?" If so, where does it go?

Some chiropractors suggest that it is your bones that go out of alignment. That may be true but the key question is "what is causing the misalignment?" If you've been paying attention you know by now that, typically, it's the muscle imbalances and tight, short muscles in spasm pulling everything, including your bones, out of alignment and creating painful trigger points.

Muscles move your bones, bones don't move muscles,

Tight muscles pull you out of alignment in all different directions. If anything is thrown out, it is your muscles that are responsible.

The expression "my back just went out," is a bit like saying the lights just went out. There's an electrical or power problem. In which case, you don't need to replace all the bulbs in the now darkened lights. Remember, good adaptation is about the right sequence. So, check the fuse box first and work out why the power is out. Get to the cause of the problem rather than focusing on the immediate effect/symptom.

So, no, your back is going nowhere. In truth, it's all locked up and couldn't go anywhere even if it had to. When, finally, your body reaches its pain threshold and it seems like it's "going out," the reality is that your muscles and soft-tissues are so tight and out of balance that they have destroyed your alignment causing the landmine knots called trigger points.

There can be a fine line between excruciating pain and mild discomfort. Many of my clients have told me on their first visit that they think they are fine with manageable discomfort but they are, in reality, only a slight movement away from crossing that threshold and reaching for the painkillers. The truth is that they are living just below the pain threshold. The slightest movement, reaching down for something or even an action as simple as brushing teeth, can increase the muscle imbalance and the intensity of the knots and trigger points, leading to a massive escalation in pain.

Often people will say something like "I reached down and that was the straw that broke the camel's back." Of course, a camel has two backs, which might help them get over the hump. However, we humans only have one and we need to protect it and treat it effectively. And part of that is to realize that our muscle imbalances, knots and trigger points might be just one small movement away from rendering us immobile.

Another expression to describe these dynamics is to say and think that, "my back gets locked up." Your back is not a criminal, even though at times it feels like a straightjacket of muscle spasm "locking" you up. Yes, you might feel like you can't move, and you can't, but it's not your back's fault. It's those muscle knots and trigger points that are putting you in a prison of pain and immobility.

The message: An ounce of prevention is worth a pound of cure. We need to be pro-active and take care of our muscles before they start complaining. There's no time like the present, and there's no present better than giving yourself the gift of movement and a pain-free life.

MYTH #4: SITTING IS A PERFECTLY NORMAL ACTIVITY

We think that sitting is a normal activity and in some ways it is. However, it's not just sitting that's the problem, it's sitting for hours on end without moving that's the problem.

For most of human history, movement was much more prevalent than sitting. However, in the last hundred years, and especially with the development of technology, sitting has reached unprecedented levels. The desk worker has been here for a mere speck of human existence.

The fact is that we were not designed to sit all day. It's an unnatural position for a long period of time during which our muscles atrophy and effectively "shut down."

This is what happens to astronauts when they are in low or no gravity environments. We need to move and our muscles weaken when they are not used. That's the gravity of the situation.

MYTH #5: DOING NOTHING IS FINE IF MY BACK PAIN GOES AWAY

Do you find it hard to take action for your back and neck pain, other than popping a pill in hopes it just goes away? This is the daily cycle and epidemic for millions of pain sufferers subjecting their bodies to harmful pharmaceuticals without taking further action to get to the cause of their pain and eliminating it for good. The pain is nothing more than a message to you and your body saying I need some help here. Listen to the message, avoid just sweeping it under the rug, otherwise the pain will never truly go away.

CHAPTER FIVE

WHY MOST TREATMENTS AND METHODS FAIL

Let's recap the critical issues.

As explained in Myth #1, it's scientifically proven that 90% of physical, chronic pain comes from the soft-tissues, especially the "landmine knot" trigger points and muscle spasms due to muscle imbalances inside them. However, these are rarely the targets of conventional treatments partly because health practitioners are not taught to understand this mechanism, instead going with a model of care that is focused on symptomatic relief.

So, physicians don't specialize in hands-on treatment of muscular pain and dysfunction, preferring instead to prescribe pain pills, and referring to physical therapists or surgeons. Less than approximately 3% of medical school is actually devoted to hands-on treatment of muscular-skeletal pain conditions.

Chiropractors typically prefer to manipulate your bones hoping this will have the correcting effect on soft-tissues, muscle balance, and trigger points. Physiotherapists and trainers usually emphasize strengthening exercises, ultrasound, and ice and are either unable or unwilling to treat your soft-tissues, which are the root cause. I also suspect that even when they know how, many PTs prefer not to, because doing quality soft-tissue therapy is harder work than simply directing exercises!

Acupuncturists treat meridians and energy lines, which do not address the root cause of muscle imbalances and trigger points.

In my view, bodyworkers are the closest thing to being the true "Pain Doctors" because they are the only ones who specialize in treating your muscles, trigger points, and soft-tissues hands-on.

Even then, most bodyworkers or soft-tissue therapists need better training to develop the skills which target and treat the root cause of your pain, muscle imbalances, and thoroughly release the trigger points

You can see, that while there are so many therapies and practitioners, all of whom are looking for your businesses and claiming to be your solution, they aren't all created the same.

Where will you choose to spend your precious dollars? Who will you engage to help you through this life-altering problem? This is a vital decision, so treat it like your life depends on it, because it does. It's not just your movement that is at stake, your entire health, relationships, and quality of life are.

The Problem of Cognitive Bias

Every practitioner believes that they can help you. And each practitioner obviously believes in the power of their particular therapy. This is what is called *confirmation bias*. We convince ourselves that our behavior is justified by only looking at evidence that supports our position and ignoring other evidence that suggests there are better alternatives.

While I realize that I, like all humans, are subject to the same cognitive biases, I have seen the evidence for myself. That evidence exists not just in research papers but in the relief that I have seen in my clients for more than two decades and the relief that I myself felt from these techniques. If I was just fooling myself, I would have been out of business a long time ago. Unlike the family doctor who is a jack-of-all-trades, I specialize in back and neck pain relief, and if they didn't work, I wouldn't have one of the *most successful clinics that specifically treats these issues* in Southern California.

The family physicians, the chiropractors, the physical therapists, the acupuncturists and whomever else, are applying a generally helpful principle and technique to a very specific problem. I believe you need specific therapies that are tailored to the specifics of the problem, not generalizations.

The fact is that you need to be your biggest advocate when going to different practitioners. Understand the lens through which they are looking at the problem. The internist may prescribe anti-inflammatory pills thinking its inflammation, the surgeon will likely suggest an MRI to see if you're a surgery candidate, the chiropractor will adjust your bones, the PT will likely recommend some strengthening exercises, and the acupuncturist will talk about chi blockages.

While all these practitioners have value in some situations and they might even help reduce the pain, ask yourselves, as well as them, why these generalized methods would work on your back, neck and muscular pain? Ask them how they will directly improve your muscle balance and function and get rid of pain causing trigger points. Whatever mode of therapy you choose, make sure your practitioner knows how to treat trigger points and muscle imbalances first, in order to get to the root cause of the pain.

DON'T GIVE UP, YOU HAVEN'T TRIED EVERYTHING!

It's not uncommon for many people to try what they consider to be the standard treatments because they don't know about muscle imbalances and trigger points. Having tried everything and experienced only temporary relief, many of these folks take a fatalistic position that they have done all they can and this is how they will live for the rest of their lives.

Of course, they haven't tried everything.

By reading this book, you have taken the massive and necessary step of educating yourself about the causes of, and effective treatments for, your back and neck pain.

Now you know there is a cure! Set your goal that you will get out of the pain!

At my clinic, we often see people who declare on their first visit, "I've tried everything," and are pretty pessimistic about their outcomes. They often come as a last resort, referred by friends or have discovered us on the web. More often than not our treatments end their back and neck pain for good. And they would have never found that relief without a mindset of hope.

***

CHAPTER SIX

BACK/NECK PAIN CAUSES

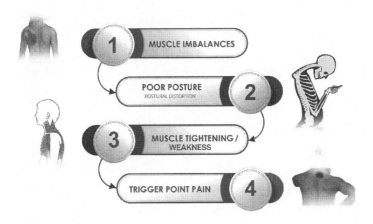

Like my successful clients I want you to be empowered by understanding the real process behind back and neck pain and the ways to effectively treat it.

Back and neck pain just don't suddenly occur. The vast percentage of the time they occur because the muscle imbalances have been accumulating over time in your body without you being aware of them. As these muscle imbalances build, certain muscles start taking over and dominating others, creating "postural distortions" and "structural misalignments" in your body. These muscle imbalances lead to poor posture, like rounded shoulders, too much tilt or rotation in your pelvis, or inefficient alignment of your neck, shoulders, hips, and knees.

We're not born to have poor posture. We're actually born with a healthy postural blueprint, yet over time muscle imbalances assaulted by the force of gravity start having their way with our posture and structure. As your posture and structure deteriorates, muscles become shorter, tighter, and weaker, and start forming trigger point knots that cause a ton of pain (Figures J and K).

Figure J

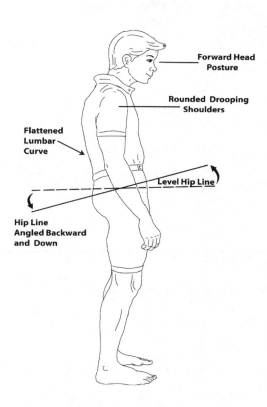

Figure K

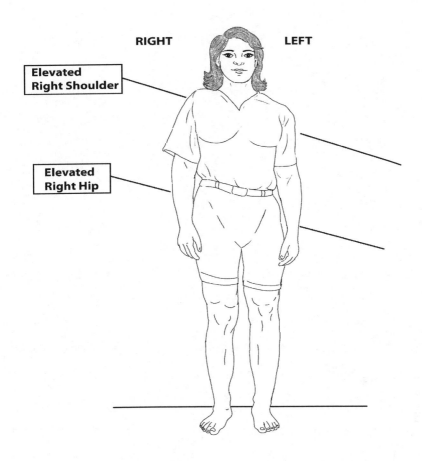

RIGHT LEFT

Elevated
Right Shoulder

Elevated
Right Hip

Do you want to finally get rid of your pain? If so, you need to first extinguish the "pain fire" trigger points and get rid of all the tight muscle spasms directly. It's the trigger point directly creating your pain, so you've got to be a good firefighter and put it out.

In STEP 1, this is the basis of the Neuromuscular Alignment System (NAS).

LISTEN TO YOUR INNER PAIN CHILD WITHIN!

Pain, like uncomfortable emotions, is often a message telling you that something is wrong and you better pay attention to it. Not just pay attention to it, but actually do something about it. You can think of pain as an inner child crying out for help. It sometimes is screaming, throwing a tantrum, pleading with you for help.

So, sure, you can take some meds, but that is simply shutting the screaming child up, not attending to the problem. He'll be screaming again soon enough. And he won't stop until he is properly fixed.

Now you don't stop a child's temper tantrum by ignoring him or her, or getting mad at the child, no matter what you might have been told by amateur psychotherapists. You solve the temper tantrum by showing the child attention, love and compassion. That doesn't mean you give him everything he demands but it does mean you treat him with love and compassion.

I say that not just out of some feel-good principle but from a biological perspective.

What happens if you get mad at your body, mad at your pain, deeply frustrated with your situation? Well, your primitive brain goes into gear, and creates the typical fight/flight responses, which when prolonged, sends hormones and cortisol throughout your body. And what do they do? They ramp up inflammation!

Now, you may know that cortisol is designed to decrease inflammation, but under continual stress, the cortisol response is compromised and instead of reducing inflammation, it actually creates it.

Getting mad at your pain only makes it worse biologically.

What happens if you treat your body and your self with love and compassion? Well, instead of releasing inflammatory chemicals, you produce anti-inflammatory and pain-reducing ones, like oxytocin and endorphins. The literature is full of research and stories about how love and compassion are truly and biologically healing. From David Spiegel's work at Stanford that showed cancer patients in support groups survived longer and had better quality lives, to cardiologist Dean Ornish's claim that the best cure for heart disease is love and compassion, there's compelling evidence that being kind to yourself and others is the best way of staying healthy.

Have self-compassion for that hurting child within, especially if there's real anger, trauma, and suffering. Put it into perspective and remember that although getting mad, frustrated and stressed seems only natural, it is actually hurting you. Be compassionate to others but most of all be compassionate with yourself. And, the healthier you are physically, without chronic pain, without suffering, the more compassionate, empathetic, and able to service others you are. Once

73

you tend to that hurting voice within though, and the physical chronic pain continues, the following steps are needed in order to get rid of it for good.

Now, before you continue I want to reinforce my message as told by Dr. David Hanscom, a spinal surgeon. He says the following:

"If you're considering having spinal surgery as the final fix for your back pain, I'd like to help you to think again about your options.

"I'm a spinal surgeon and I want you to know that surgery is not your best option for recovery from low back pain."

Dr. Hanscom lists three reasons for not having surgery.

"1. Surgery for relieving back pain has never been shown to be effective in a stringent research study. The most careful research paper published in 2006 demonstrated that only 22% of patients were satisfied with the outcomes two years later. Essentially, all research shows consistently poor outcomes for fusion surgery performed for back pain."

"The first reason to avoid fusion surgery is that it simply doesn't work. It isn't even indicated. It's very difficult for anyone to identify the exact source of back pain. We can be confident only about 5-10% of the time. We also know that disc degeneration, ruptured discs, bulging discs, arthritis, and narrowed discs have been clearly shown to NOT be the source of chronic back pain. Yet these changes are the most common reason that surgery is suggested. A high percentage of people without any back pain have various disc disorders and by age 65 it reaches 100%."

2. "Secondly, several studies have shown that if surgery is performed in any part of the body in the presence of ongoing chronic pain, it can induce chronic pain at the new surgical site up to 60% of the time. In other words, if you are suffering from chronic neck pain and undergo a hernia repair, you can develop ongoing groin pain and it can be permanent 5-10% of the time. Normally a hernia operation is almost painless. If I had a neurological complication rate this high, I couldn't remain in practice."

3. "The final reason for not considering surgery for back pain is that chronic back pain can be reliably solved with the correct treatment approaches."

There you have it from a spinal surgeon.

Now let's focus on what will work.

***

CHAPTER SEVEN

BACK PAIN RELIEF SECRETS REVEALED!

THE 5 STEP SOLUTION TO BE PAIN-FREE!

As you have read so far, there is new hope for back and neck pain sufferers tired of living in pain. With the understanding of those landmine knot trigger points and muscle imbalances, we have finally got to the point where we can find relief, moreover long-term relief that fixes the problem. Unfortunately, not everyone in practice understands that yet, but those that do are able to provide long-lasting solutions.

The following explains why doing therapy and engaging different treatment modalities in the wrong order and sequence (e.g. strengthening muscles too soon) is a recipe for disaster. The order of therapeutic techniques is very important to get rid of your pain. Doing them out of order often leads to increased pain, inflammation and a worsening of your situation. For example, doing strengthening exercises too soon in an inflamed painful area often increases pain.

The Secret to Making Your Back and Neck Pain Permanently Disappear is the SEQUENCE of Therapy!

I am about to describe the five steps that need to be done in the right sequence. Our exclusive NAS Therapy method of neuromuscular trigger point therapy, postural alignment therapy, and restoring muscle balance and function are the crucial first three steps.

The fact is that the order in which you do therapeutic techniques is crucial to curing your back/neck pain for good and for proper rehabilitation of injured soft tissues

STEP #1: NEUROMUSCULAR/TRIGGER POINT THERAPY (NAS THERAPY) FOR INSTANT RELIEF!

Have you ever noticed how you can stretch, strengthen, take pills, meditate, pray, and try every single thing in the book, yet your back and neck pain never goes away? That's because over 90%+ of chronic pain comes from pain-causing trigger points in the soft-tissues, and nothing gets rid of these landmine knots except for manual, hands-on direct pressure by a highly skilled practitioner and method, such as our NAS Therapy method. The other option, less effective than a practitioner yet still very powerful, is learning how to self-treat and release your own trigger points in your body.

You can stretch all day long, go on a week long yoga retreat, get adjusted 5 days a week for months on end by a chiropractor, do the most elite physical therapy exercises in the world, yet none of these methods will get rid of the painful trigger points causing your pain. Trigger points won't release from just stretching, strengthening, adjusting, ice, heat, or ultrasound.

Getting rid of muscle spasms, hyper-contractions, and trigger points in the soft-tissues is your most important first step.

If simply "loose muscles," stretching, and flexibility were the answers, then why do we see so many yoga students and teachers, gymnasts, and ballet dancers with so much back and neck pain?

Become Your Own Firefighter!

PUT THE FIRE OUT FIRST, BE A "FIREFIGHTER"

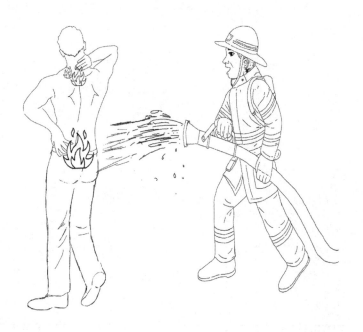

Becoming a "firefighter" is the very first stage of rehabilitation to get rid of the hyper-constricted soft-tissues and muscle spasms and pain causing trigger points!

When you're in pain, you just want it gone. It's like a fire you just want to put out. It's crucial to put out the source of the pain "fire" first, and eliminate those landmine knot trigger points creating all the discomfort.

That's why highly skilled bodywork and soft-tissue therapy is so important, so you attack your pain on all levels, and like a firefighter you put out the "pain flame" with advanced forms of therapeutic treatments. Only once you put out the flame, are you able to get closer to the source of it and put that out too. The other main sources are muscle imbalances, structural misalignments, and postural distortions, yet you must first squash that "pain flame" and get rid of the muscle spasms and trigger points FIRST, before moving on to the other steps.

Again, direct pressure by a practitioner or yourself is the most effective way to de-activate those painful trigger point landmine knots. It's the first line of defense to fight pain for good and stop it. And the best way to defuse the landmine knots and put out the pain is manually, through effective hands-on therapy by a highly skilled bodyworker in our exclusive NAS Method. This can be supplemented through self-treatment with certain massage tools, balls and foam rollers.

You can call our back and neck relief NAS experts here in Los Angeles (www.MassageRevolution.com) or try finding someone near you. Either way, our staff is here to support you with any questions you may have.

Now, in the interests of accuracy, high quality instruction and helping you the most, I am not going to show you photos of what you need to do because photos are easy to misunderstand and don't convey the important movement dynamics that are critical for understanding and ultimate success. I make no apologies for directing you to videos of these exercises, which convey the *movement* necessary for success.

5 SIMPLE WAYS TO SELF-TREAT YOUR OWN TRIGGER POINTS AT HOME FOR BACK/NECK PAIN RELIEF!

Be sure to watch the free videos I created for the "5 Simple Ways To Self-Treat Your Own Trigger Points At Home For Back/Neck Pain Relief"

www.MassageRevolution.com/BackNeckReliefVideos.html

These videos show you how to self-treat your own back and neck muscles and trigger points at home, to help you put out that "pain flame" and give you instant, lasting pain relief right at the source.

STEP 2: RESTORE PROPER MUSCLE BALANCE AND FUNCTION, CORRECT POOR POSTURE AND BIOMECHANICS, WITH NAS THERAPY

NAS Therapy accomplishes a few things. It releases trigger points to get rid of the "pain flame" and additionally fixes muscle imbalances and postural dysfunctions in several different ways.

First, NAS Therapy greatly improves your muscle balance by the NAS practitioner releasing your over-dominating short, tight muscles in a very detailed and specific way. This brings your muscles and body back into balance and better alignment.

Second, NAS Therapy greatly restores proper muscle balance with specific muscle balancing exercises. Once the NAS therapist releases your trigger points, and the muscle spasms are gone, you implement unique muscle balance exercises specific and unique to your body's alignment, to make a huge effect on getting rid of your pain for good.

Imagine for a moment your body is like a mold of clay, and you can shape it any way you wish. With Step 1 above you're first shaping the muscles and body by releasing all the spasms and hyper-constrictions so they all become smooth and in proper alignment.

Now that you've set your body's postural "mold" in place, will it just stick and stay there? No! You need some sort of "glue" so your new body, posture, muscle balance retains its shape, and postural muscle balance exercises are exactly that. NAS Therapy provides specific muscle balance exercises as the "glue" to retain the benefits of Step 1 above.

Be sure to watch the free videos I created for the "9 Postural Alignment Exercises To Fix Your Own Muscle Imbalances At Home For Back/Neck Pain Relief"

www.MassageRevolution.com/BackNeckReliefVideos.html

These exercises are shown in the video and <u>must</u> be done in the following sequence and order.

1. Gluteal Squeezes
2. Bent Knee Squeezes
3. Inner Thigh Stretch
4. Reverse Pressing
5. Side Lateral Raises
6. Hip Opener
7. Hip Crossover
8. Flexion/Extension
9. Wall Sit

STEP #3 RESTORE FLEXIBILITY TO THE SOFT-TISSUES (STRETCHING)

REMINDER: YOU MUST LENGTHEN BEFORE YOU STRENGTHEN!

As mentioned previously, people often stretch for years without increasing any mobility or decreasing their pain. That truly is the definition of insanity, doing the same thing over and over again yet expecting a different result (as per Albert Einstein).

Trigger points often shut down muscles making them impossible to stretch. It's often only when you implement Step 1 above and finally release the trigger points in the muscle belly, that you are then able to finally stretch out the muscle. And when your muscles are in a constant state of war and power struggle, it's difficult to stretch as well. Proper muscle balance exercises in Step 2, bring more peace and balance to your muscles, and now stretching is finally more productive. Without proper muscle balance exercises first and the muscle neurologically "firing" correctly, the stretching often goes to waste.

Once you have the highly skilled NAS bodyworker first release your trigger points or you self-treat them at home, to get rid of the "pain flame," fix poor posture habits, and you restore proper muscle balance so muscles engage better, notice how much more effective your stretches are.

THE SECRET FOR HOW TO GET A MUCH BETTER STRETCH! TREAT TRIGGER POINTS RIGHT BEFORE YOU STRETCH!

To get the most out of your stretch, treat and release the trigger points in that muscle first (Step 1 above) right before you stretch that muscle. Releasing the trigger points first is like releasing the "lock" on your muscle to free it up and allow it to actually stretch much better!

Be sure to watch the free videos I created for the "Top 5 Stretches To Treat And Relieve Your Own Back/Neck Pain At Home."

www.MassageRevolution.com/BackNeckReliefVideos.html

STEP 4: REBUILD THE STRENGTH OF THE INJURED SOFT-TISSUES THROUGH RESISTANCE TRAINING!

Once you get rid of the trigger points, restore proper muscle balance and flexibility to the painful and/or injured soft-tissues (Steps 1-3), it's time to rebuild the strength of the injured tissues with resistance training. Doing this too soon runs the risk of re-injuring and flaring up an already inflamed painful region. The key is to do more bodyweight functional exercises and progress to strength training exercises such as kettlebells, not machines that lock your body, structure and joints in a fixed position.

> Be sure to watch the free videos I created for the "5 Simple Ways to Strengthen For Back/Neck Pain Relief."
>
> www.MassageRevolution.com/BackNeckReliefVideos.html

STEP 5: REBUILD ENDURANCE (AEROBIC EXERCISES)

Dynamic, functional exercises that rebuild your body's endurance are an important final step when rehabilitating from back and neck pain. When you have healthy muscle balance and function, minimal pain, and you are strong, stable, and balanced with your postural stabilizer muscles, more vigorous endurance exercises are great. A functional body is meant for activities such as brisk walking, sprinting, hiking, swimming, biking, and more.

It is important NOT to use a treadmill for the aerobic, endurance exercises. When you use a treadmill, the machine itself naturally pulls your legs backwards, which means that your gluteal muscles don't have to naturally do that and prevents them from engaging properly. The treadmill is doing the work, instead of your gluteals. As a result, the treadmill is creating an unnatural movement which is not effective training. You need to be training all the muscles to be doing their job, and this doesn't happen on the treadmill.

***

CHAPTER EIGHT

GETTING STARTED: YOUR PAIN RELIEF ACTION PLANS

8 WEEK FREEDOM FROM BACK & NECK PAIN ACTION PLAN

WEEKS 1-2: (Month 1)

1. Seek out a highly skilled NAS Therapist (Neuromuscular Alignment Specialist) to treat your trigger points and muscle imbalances 2 times per week for 4 weeks. (STEP 1)

   Feel free to call our staff for any questions or support (www.MassageRevolution.com).

2. 15-30 minutes per day self-treatment trigger points (STEP 1). Have your NAS Therapist show you the exact trigger points you must release and self-treat at home to be pain-free!

3. Implement daily all of the "Top 10 Lifestyle Changes To Enjoy A Pain-Free Life" (see page 89).

WEEKS 3-4: (Month 1)

1. Continue NAS Therapy twice per week. (STEP 1)

2. Continue 15-30 minutes per day self-treatment trigger points (STEP 1).

3. Continue to implement daily all of the "Top 10 Lifestyle Changes To Enjoy A Pain-Free Life" (see page 89).

4. START 20-30 minutes per day (at least 5 days per week) of Muscle Balance Exercises (STEP 2)

WEEKS 5-6: (Month 2)

1. Continue 20-30 minutes per day Muscle Balance Exercises (STEP 2).

2. Continue NAS Therapy 1-2 times per month.

3. Continue 15 minutes for 3 days per week self-treatment trigger points (STEP 1).

4. START 10 minutes stretching (STEP 3) right after self-treatment of trigger points (STEP 1).

5. Continue to implement daily all of the "Top 10 Lifestyle Changes To Enjoy A Pain-Free Life" (see page 89).

WEEKS 7-8: (Month 2)

1. Continue 20-30 minutes per day Muscle Balance Exercises (STEP 2).

2. Continue NAS Therapy 1-2 times per month.

3. Continue 15 minutes for 3 days per week self-treatment trigger points (STEP 1).

4. Continue 10 minutes stretching (STEP 3) right after self-treatment of trigger points (STEP 1).

5. START 15 minutes/day, 3 days/week bodyweight functional strengthening exercises (STEP 4), with no pain.

6. Continue to implement daily all of the "Top 10 Lifestyle Changes To Enjoy A Pain-Free Life"

TOP 10 LIFESTYLE CHANGES TO ENJOY A PAIN-FREE LIFE!

1. Walking 15-30 minutes a day is the best activity overall for healthy muscle balance and function, as our #1 main function is movement. It's best for "engaging" and activating the gluteal muscles and postural/pelvic stabilizer muscles in the most functional way possible. Avoid the treadmill, as it's much less of a functional movement and hinders the "engaging" of postural muscles due to the moving floor pulling your legs backward and hijacking the work for you.

2. How To Walk Correctly! To walk correctly, your feet need to be pointed straight forward, with your ankles, knees and shoulders also pointed straight ahead. Do not lead with your head. Remember every inch that your head is forward of your body, adds an extra 10 pounds of pull on your neck. So, align your feet, knees, hips and shoulders, and your ears over your shoulders. Your arms should swing in parallel to your body, not across your body. Think of a soldier marching;

soldiers keep their arms moving in the forward plane without deviating from it. You can try this out and see what happens when your arms swing across your body instead of straight forward. Notice how the shoulders and neck get pulled out of alignment.

3. How To Sit Correctly At Your Desk! The middle of your computer screen must be at eye level for proper neck/shoulder alignment and muscle balance. Take a 5 min walk every hour. Remember, sitting causes your pelvic, gluteal and postural stabilizing muscles to atrophy and fall asleep, so getting up regularly for a walk keeps those muscles engaging and activating properly.

4. How To Stand Correctly! You stand correctly by having equal weight on both feet. Your feet are not wide apart but parallel and pointing straight ahead hip width apart. Your knees, hips, shoulders are aligned with your ears aligned with your shoulders, so your head is not leaning forward.

5. How To Sleep Correctly! For optimal alignment and muscle balance, sleep on your back, like "corpse pose" in yoga! Use just a small pillow, nothing too thick to avoid lifting your head/neck too high out of alignment. Sleeping on your side or stomach creates muscle imbalances and trigger points in your back, neck, hips. If you must be a side-sleeper, put a pillow between your knees and under your top arm. Avoid stomach sleeping at all costs!

6. How To Breath Correctly! Abdominal, diaphragm, and "belly breathing" instead of "chest breathing" is the most natural form of breathing, just watch how babies and toddlers breath. Lie down for a minute, put one hand on your upper chest and sternum, the other right above your pubic bone, and notice which hand moves the most as you inhale and exhale. Ideally, just your lower hand is moving mainly, as this oxygenates and energizes your cells optimally. The benefits for your back and neck of this type of breathing are immense. It relaxes your back and neck muscles, calms your nervous system, to enable your muscles to finally let go and be pain-free!

7. Release all anger and resentments: All anger and resentments do to your back and neck is cause a "burning" of your muscles, fascia, and soft-tissues, locking you into and exacerbating the pain-spasm cycle. Stop the cycle and stop the pain! Remind yourself that we as humans are mistake makers by nature and nobody is perfect, so forgive yourself and those who have hurt you, let it go, you're only hurting yourself. Each morning/evening write in your gratitude journal, daily forgiving yourself for all self-judgments. Breathe correctly in your abdomen (belly breathing)

8. Mental Rehearsal:, Do 3 min/day on your self image, imagining yourself PAIN-FREE. Why? Because "You can't outperform your self-image" and if you're constantly

imagining yourself as a "back pain sufferer" then that's what you are. As Dennis Waitley says, "Your mental images are your previews of your life's coming attractions."

Research has constantly shown that visualization is practice. Your brain doesn't distinguish between reality and imagination. Visualization isn't just a reminder, it's real life practice which facilitates doing the exercises needed to get your life back. You truly do become what you think about most of the time, so why not imagine yourself pain-free more. What does it look like? What do you look like? What activities are you doing? How do you feel? Visual it all!

9. Eating: Low inflammation diet, an anti-inflammatory diet. No refined sugar, dairy. Lean meats, healthy proteins, lots of veggies.
10. Water: Dehydration deprives your body and muscles of required electrolytes…Drink lots of water, hydrate your cells.

WHY YOU MUST TAKE RESPONSIBILITY

"You are 100% responsible for your life!" – Brian Tracy

Have you noticed some days are better than others with regards to your pain? Do you ever ask yourself why this is, yet find it impossible to figure out? Is your pain less on days you are happier? When you repeat the mantra "I am 100% responsible for my life" over and over to yourself, more often than not you feel more in control of your life. When you feel more in control of your life, you feel happier, more peaceful, less resentful. More happiness and peace, less anger and resentment, is a GREAT recipe for helping to get rid of your pain. There's a huge mind-body connection with regards to your pain, and being more mindful of this leads you much further along your path to recovery. You have a choice every morning you wake up. You can choose to say to yourself that you are 100% responsible for your life, and feel more empowered and in control.

Use the daily reminders to practice getting your muscles released, your posture aligned and your soul freed up!

The longer you wait the worse it will get.

Take charge of your pain, now!

***

References

Chapter 1

Chou R, Shekelle P. Will this Patient Develop Persistent Disabling Low Back Pain? Journal of the American Medical Association. 2010; 303(13):1295-1302.

Haiou Y, Haldeman, S., Ming-Lun L, & Baker, D. Low Back Pain Prevalence and Related Workplace Psychosocial Risk Factors: A Study Using Data From the 2010 National Health Interview SurveyJ Manipulative Physiol Ther. 2016 September ; 39(7): 459–472.

Chapter 3

Kripke DF, Garfinkel L, Wingard DL, Klauber MR, Marler MR (2002). Mortality associated with sleep duration and insomnia. Arch Gen Psychiatry. 2002;59:131–6

Tamakoshi A, & Ohno Y. (2004). Self-reported sleep duration as a predictor of all-cause mortality: results from the JACC study, Japan. Sleep. 2004;27:51–4

Benito-Leon J, Bermejo-Pareja F, Vega S et al. (2009) Total daily sleep duration and the risk of dementia: A prospective population-based study. Eur J Neurol 2009;16:990–997.

Foley DJ, Monjan AA, Masaki KH et al. (1999) Associations of symptoms of sleep apnea with cardiovascular disease, cognitive impairment, and mortality among elderly Japanese-American men. J Am Geriatr Soc 1999;47:524–528.

Sarno,J. (1998) The Mind-Body Prescription: Healing the Body, Healing the Mind. Warner books, New York.

H. Pentikäinen, K. Savonen, P. Komulainen, V. Kiviniemi, T. Paajanen, M. Kivipelto, H. Soininen, R. Rauramaa. (2017) Muscle strength and cognition in ageing men and women: The DR's EXTRA study. European Geriatric Medicine, 2017; 8 (3):

Wheaton AG, Chapman DP, Presley-Cantrell LR, Croft JB, Roehler DR. Drowsy driving – 19 states and the District of Columbia, 2009-2010. Cdc-pdf. MMWR Morb Mortal Wkly Rep. 2013; 61:1033.

Wheaton AG, Shults RA, Chapman DP, Ford ES, Croft JB. Drowsy driving and risk behaviors—10 states and Puerto Rico, 2011-2012. Cdc-pdf MMWR Morb Mortal Wkly Rep. 2014; 63:557-562.

Chapter 5

Kahneman, D. (2013). Thinking, fast and slow, Farrar, Straus and Giroux

Chapter 6

Dean Ornish (1999). Love and Survival: The scientific basis of the healing power of intimacy. Harper Collins

Hanscom, D. (2016) Back in Control. Vertus Press.

Spiegel, D. & Classen, C. (2001) Group Therapy for Cancer Patients: a Research-Based Handbook of Psychosocial Care: A Research-Based Handbook of Psychosocial Care. Basic Books

Acknowledgements

Most importantly, this book is dedicated to all those who suffer with chronic pain in hope for a solution for lasting relief.

I'm truly honored and forever grateful for all the clients who've entrusted me with their care.

To my amazing team at The Back & Neck Relief Center, committed to our mission as the leading soft-tissue center for more serious pain relief, helping chronic pain sufferers live healthier and pain-free, without surgery and pharmaceuticals.

I am extremely grateful and appreciative for the love and support of my family. They always provide me the inspiration and courage to dream big, that everything is possible.

Dear Reader:

I want to thank you, one for getting this book, and two, for actually taking the time to read it.

Investing time and money into your own health and self-improvement is one of the best investments you can make. The final, most important decision you now must make is to act on what you've discovered inside these pages. And that doesn't necessarily mean coming into our clinic to see our back and neck pain relief experts.

Sure, I'd love for you to come see us so we're able to help you get rid of your back and neck pains, or other aches and pains for good, but at the end of the day, whether it's with us, on your own, or with someone else, I hope you just ACT and TAKE ACTION.

This can be the end or a grand beginning of a healthier, pain-free life for you. If you found value here, and, hopefully found the information to be interesting and engaging, well, there's a lot more where this came from.

By now acting on the 5 steps outlined in the book, you're well on your way to enjoying a more pain-free, active lifestyle.

Practicing in the L.A. area and offering my unique Neuromuscular Alignment System, I have helped many famous people, from Hollywood icons to sports stars, get rid of their back and neck issues. You can get the same treatment because everyone gets celebrity treatment at The Back and Neck Relief Center.

So, if you happen to live in the Los Angeles area, and want further help from our Neuromuscular Specialists and Back/Neck Relief Experts, **just call us at 310-798-4263.**

For more information on The Back & Neck Relief Center (Massage Revolution), visit www.MassageRevolution.com.

For contacting Michael, email <u>Michael@MassageRevolution.com</u>

Special Offers!
The Best Bodywork For Serious Back and Neck Pain Relief!

The Back & Neck Relief Center
Tired of living in pain? Get rid of your pain now and call our clinic at 310-798-4263 for a new client introductory treatment!

Wellness Practice Business Coaching
Are you a wellness practitioner or business looking to grow your practice? Contact Michael for a free coaching consultation.

Workplace Consulting
Do you work for a small to large sized company who may be interested in improving workplace productivity, ergonomics, lessen work related injuries? Michael is an experienced health coach and speaker. If you're interested in booking Michael for a lecture, health talk or for workplace ergonomic consulting, please call the main office number, mention this book, and Michael will provide a free phone or in person consultation to discuss your needs.

Main Office Location:
500 S. Sepulveda Blvd Suite 101, Manhattan Beach, CA   90266

MISSION STATEMENT
To provide the most effective evidence-based bodywork for more serious pain relief, helping people move better, feel better, and live pain-free, without surgery and pharmaceuticals.

VISION STATEMENT
The Back & Neck Relief Center is the USA's leading bodywork center for serious pain relief, helping as many people as possible move better, feel better, and live pain-free, without surgery and pharmaceuticals.

CORE PURPOSE
To help chronic pain sufferers live pain-free, move better, feel better, without drugs or surgery.

About Michael Greenspan

Michael Greenspan, Neuromuscular Alignment Specialist (NAS) for 27+ years, is a leading expert in acute and chronic muscular pain relief in the fields of Neuromuscular Therapy, Kinesiology, Corrective Exercise and Biomechanics. Michael's unique holistic approach to treatment and education has changed the lives of countless clients, students and peers. By treating the body as a whole system, Michael successfully excels at getting to the root cause of clients' pain where traditional approaches have consistently failed.

SPECIALIZED TRAINING TO GET THE CARE YOU DESERVE

Michael's constant search for knowledge in the cutting edge in effective muscle and sports therapy enables him to get to the source of people's pain and finally give clients the relief they need and deserve. He utilizes NAS, corrective functional exercises and Kinesiology, active dynamic stretching, joint mobilization, core stabilization exercises, movement therapy and other techniques to offer clients a broad range of therapeutic modalities so they stay active, sit comfortably all day, move better, feel better, live pain-free, and maintain their muscles in an optimum state of relaxation—all naturally without any drugs or side effects.

A Foundation You Can Trust

Michael is highly qualified as a Neuromuscular Alignment Specialist, instructor and educator of NAS, with his degree in Kinesiology/Exercise Physiology at the University of Colorado, Boulder. He's an educator, speaker and consultant, with his life purpose to help and serve others to achieve a pain-free life.

Business Coaching

Michael's also passionate about coaching other wellness practitioners and entrepreneurs to achieve a highly successful practice quickly and easily.

More Testimonials

"I can't thank the terrific therapists at The Back and Neck Relief Center enough. With the pain I was living with for over two years, getting relief at The Back and Neck Relief Center was the only thing that kept me going through my other treatments, and now I'm feeling so much better and happier." - Becky Chao, Redondo Beach

"I feel so much better after I get a treatment here at The Back and Neck Relief Center. I come every other week to relieve my chronic neck and shoulder pain. I must have gotten a treatment from everyone here and everyone is wonderful! Thank you!!" - Jamie Sun

"Alleviated back, neck, shoulder and knee pains caused from two different car accidents." - David Gatlin, Los Angeles/Redondo Beach

"I started The Back and Neck Relief Center in 2015. For approximately three months, I had a really stiff neck from all the tension carried in my neck and shoulders. I couldn't turn my head to look to the left. I had a hard time driving because I couldn't turn my head. Within the first month of treatment, I could see a big improvement in the stiffness of my neck and shoulders. The treatments really helped me with my neck issues. I feel wonderful every time I leave after my treatment!" -Anonymous Client, Torrance

"I started at The Back and Neck Relief Center in August 2018 with pain in my right hip that wrapped around to my groin that lasted for 6 years. I saw 4 doctors and took lots of Advil. I was able to do things, but always in pain. Also, the pain interrupted my sleep. After 4 treatments at Back and Neck Pain Relief Center, results became apparent. I have increased my mobility in my hip. I have less pain overall and better sleep. I finally feel like I'm going to be totally healed." - Imoye Francis, Los Angeles

"I started The Back and Neck Relief Center circa 2016 or 2017, for back problems, anxiety, and sleep problems I had for over 2 years. I saw 4-5 doctors and received leg and back injections, but the pain was still making it difficult to get up and down, and sleep was difficult. After 4+ visits, results became apparent. It made the pain more bearable- I needed less time with doctors, less injections in my back or thigh. I was not aware these treatments are now being accepted as a non-drug, non-surgery alternative for varieties of pain." - Barry Solomon, RPH, M. Ed.

"I started at The Back and Neck Relief Center in June 2017 for lower back/neck pain, IT band problems, I had for 5 years. I went to 2-3 doctors for this. The pain used to be severe enough that I couldn't do my normal daily routine. It was approximately 1-2 months of treatments before results became apparent. I have been very impressed with the care I have received here. My pain level has gotten better. The therapists here are fantastic. There are different

therapists that specialize in different types of treatments, so there are many treatment options." - Lauren Braman, Torrance

"I started at The Back and Neck Relief Center 1/17/19 for back tightness and pain, tried ibuprofen, yet took 1 treatment before results became apparent. The Therapist was incredible, life changing! I will be back!" -- Kelley Johnson, Manhattan Beach

"I started coming October 2017 for neck and shoulder pain I was having for 1 year. I noticed very soon after results! The Back and Neck Relief Center has had a great impact on my health." - Kathy Mota, Los Angeles

"I started at The Back and Neck Relief Center in November 2017 to treat my shoulder and back pain that I experienced for 5 years. I saw two other doctors for this, but my life was interrupted a moderate amount at work. After only two months of treatment at The Back and Neck Relief Center, results became apparent. I had a great impression! They relieved my pain and helped from getting surgery." - P. Cloud, Los Angeles

Made in the USA
Columbia, SC
31 October 2021